WHY DOES SEX HURT?

A Women's Guide to Eliminating Painful Sex for Good

WHY DOES SEX HURT?

A Women's Guide to Eliminating Painful Sex for Good

J. NICOLE EISENBROWN, MD

Niche Pressworks
INDIANAPOLIS, IN

Why Does Sex Hurt?

ISBN-13: 978-1-952654-12-1 (paperback)
978-1-952654-13-8 (ebook)

Published by Niche Pressworks; http://NichePressworks.com

The information provided in this book is meant to educate the reader on the subjects discussed. It is not meant to be a substitute for medical advice, diagnosis, or treatment. Always consult your physician or other qualified health care professional to obtain help with any medically related questions or conditions.

CONTENTS

PREFACE

DOCTORS CAN ONLY TREAT WHAT THEY KNOW

WELL, FIRST OF ALL, LET'S BE HONEST. Female sexual issues, as a whole, are not taken very seriously in our society and have largely been ignored by the medical community. The field of female sexual dysfunction (which includes dyspareunia: painful intercourse) is relatively new. Gynecologists and urologists, the two specialties that deal with the male and female sexual organs, get very little, if any, training on female sexual dysfunction (FSD).

I am board certified in both urology and female pelvic medicine and reconstructive surgery (FPM-RS). But I had to seek out separate training to learn more about female sexual health. This instruction has come primarily through courses given by the American Urological Association (AUA) and the International Society for the Study of Women's Sexual

Health (ISSWSH). I've also completed multiple preceptorships with world-renowned sexual medicine experts.

While there are opportunities to learn more about FSD after training, most physicians have only a limited amount of time when they are actively in practice. So, try not to be angry or frustrated if your gynecologist is unable to help you. She can only fix what she has been trained to fix. But this does not mean that you can't get help. My goal is to help you help yourself as much as possible. If you cannot fix the problem on your own, I will help you locate a doctor in your area who has trained specifically in FSD. One of the best resources for this is ISSWSH. You can go to the ISSWSH website and look at its directory to locate a specialist near you—www1.statusplus.net/sp/isswsh/find-a-provider/.

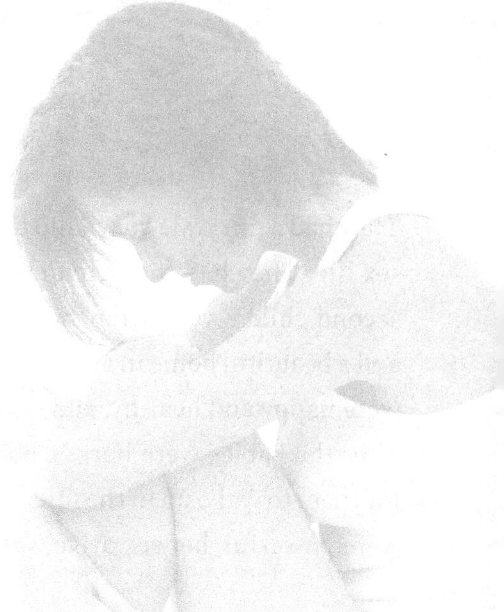

INTRODUCTION

A CRUEL JOKE

IT SEEMS LIKE A CRUEL JOKE, BUT NO ONE IS LAUGHING. You once had an amazing sex life, and then, all of a sudden, it's taken from you—like you're being punished for something you did not even know you had done!

That was how Debbie felt when I first met her. She is a wonderful forty-five-year-old woman with a very full life, happily married to David with two young boys. Debbie remembers wondering if she would ever get married or have children, but then she met David. They both believed they would meet their soulmates and had never compromised in a relationship. She and her husband had married a little later in life at the age of thirty-five, but it had still been the first marriage for both, and neither had any children.

They had a fairytale courtship that included a very active and fulfilling sex life. They had their first child two years after marrying and their second child a year after that. They each had very successful careers and a beautiful home in an upscale neighborhood. Both of their children were happy and healthy, and their sex life remained very active—even after the babies were born. Debbie recalls that it was not uncommon for them to wake up in the middle of the night to have sex! Her orgasms were powerful, her sex drive was amazing, and life was good.

Then something started to change. It began slowly at first, but sex started to hurt. She thought maybe it was a lubrication issue, so they tried using lubricants, but this did not help. The pain got worse over time. Debbie described it as a knife ripping her open as David penetrated her. David hated knowing that he was hurting her. Debbie went to her gynecologist, who prescribed some vaginal estrogen to help with "vaginal dryness," but this did not help either. No one seemed to know what the problem was, and no one was able to help—until Debbie came into my office.

After evaluating Debbie, we determined that she had the most common cause of sexual pain—hormonally mediated vestibulodynia. We'll talk about this later, but it is a very common condition. We started treatment and, within several weeks, her pain was completely gone. It has been two years since she was diagnosed and treated, and she remains pain-free.

Does this sound like you? If you are reading this, then there is a good chance that at least some of Debbie's story resonates with you. Eighty percent of women who have pain associated with sex have Debbie's condition, and it is highly curable—so read on! There are other causes of sexual pain, and they will be covered, too.

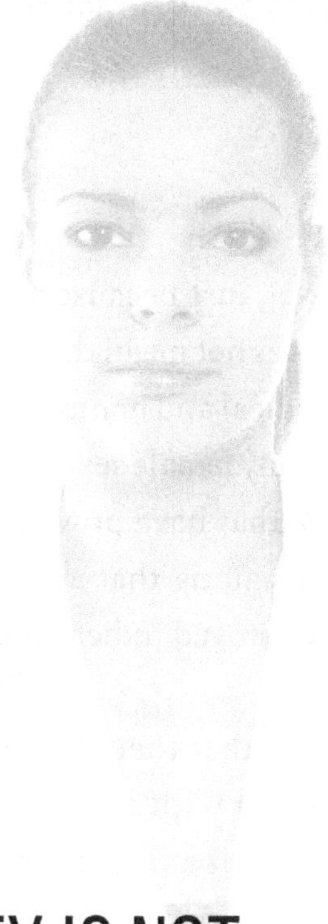

CHAPTER 1

FEMALE SEXUALITY IS NOT TAKEN SERIOUSLY

OUR SOCIETY, AS A WHOLE, does not take female sexual issues very seriously. This attitude is even prevalent in the medical community and the FDA. This fact helps explain the lack of interest, training, and research in this area. For example, until recently, the FDA had not approved any medications for women's sexual health.

Did you know that there are twenty-six FDA-approved drugs to help men with sexual dysfunction, but only one for women? Addyi, the only FDA-approved drug for female sexual function, took almost a decade to gain approval. This may sound depressing at first glance. At the very least, it is an unfortunate statement about how little our society and the medical community value the satisfaction of women.

However, just because there aren't a variety of medications to choose from does not mean these conditions are untreatable—there are numerous medical and nonmedical treatments available that can successfully treat many female sexual conditions. And in fact, there are several medications that have proven to be successful, but they must be given off label, meaning that a physician must prescribe them outside of their FDA-approved indication.

Don't let that thought scare you—many of the medications you may be familiar with are frequently prescribed off label. This is a common practice. It is a very expensive proposition to get a drug approved by the FDA, often costing pharma companies hundreds of millions of dollars. But once a drug is approved for use in one disease state, physicians can use it for other problems as well. Both the FDA and medical community understand that while a medication is usually only approved to treat one thing, many drugs have multiple uses and can be effective in treating a variety of conditions.

HOW COMMON IS PAIN WITH INTERCOURSE (DYSPAREUNIA)?

Dyspareunia, which is defined as pain with intercourse, falls under the larger topic of female sexual dysfunction, or FSD. There are several areas in which women can have difficulty: arousal, low desire, pain with penetration, and problems reaching orgasm. Each of these is very real for many women, but for the purpose of this writing, I will focus on painful intercourse. It may not be the most common of the complaints, but it is perhaps the most distressful.

Problems in the bedroom are not limited to erectile dysfunction in men. From all the ads on TV for erectile dysfunction medications, you would think that every man has this issue and that it is the only problem between the sheets. You never hear or see any information about women and their sexual problems, which is a shame. Women experience sexual problems with the same frequency as men, but they rarely get treated. Forty-four percent—almost half—of women in this country will experience some degree of sexual dysfunction in their lifetime. That is more than the incidence of high blood pressure and diabetes combined!

Approximately 20 percent of women will experience painful sex, which is often a chronic problem that can destroy relationships and do untold damage to a woman's self-esteem. It can also dramatically increase the risk of depression—many believe that depression leads to sexual dysfunction, but the opposite is also true. Women who have pain with intercourse are two and a half times as likely to be depressed as the general population, and women who are unable to reach orgasm are more than five times as likely to suffer from depression.

THE CYCLE OF PAIN

There is a vicious pain cycle that occurs with dyspareunia. If, for example, you have pain with intercourse, then it is likely that you will instinctively tighten your pelvic floor muscles before the penetration occurs. This is a protective reaction to pain and is perfectly normal. However, this can lead to pelvic floor spasms, which is, itself, another cause of pain. This only makes the problem worse, as you now have two causes of sex-related pain.

Additionally, most couples become frustrated and confused about the problem. Some women may have partners who accuse them of making it up or tell them it's all in their head. This can cause guilt and shame and can lead to decreased self-esteem, relationship issues, and depression. Now, if you add to the mix a visit with a doctor who does not know how to help you, then you are left wondering if, in fact, you *are* crazy. Well, you are not crazy, at least not about this! (That was a joke, if you missed it!)

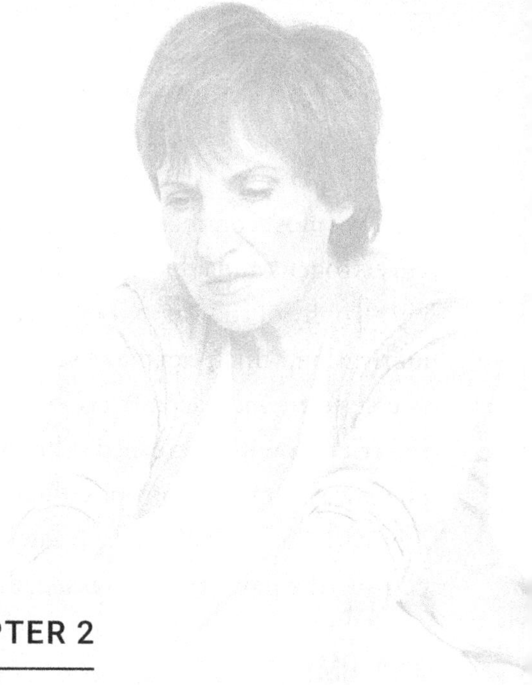

CHAPTER 2

IDENTIFYING THE CAUSE OF PAIN

OKAY, LET'S DELVE INTO THIS. Ninety-seven percent of women with sexual pain have a physiological cause for it. It is not in your head. Some doctors, unfortunately, will want to attribute dyspareunia (pain with intercourse) to sexual abuse, anxiety, or depression. Although women who have been sexually abused are more likely to experience pain with intercourse, the vast majority do not fall into this category. And even if you do, it may still be a medical problem that can be treated.

If you have seen a doctor about painful intercourse, you may have been given antibiotics or antifungals to treat an infection. Sometimes doctors will even prescribe steroids. But rarely are infections (of any type) the cause of chronic pain with intercourse, and there are only a few disorders that require steroids. Consequently, these medications often provide little or no improvement.

The two most common solutions suggested by medical doctors are vaginal estrogens and lubrication. Both are good ideas if the problem is simply atrophy of the vaginal mucosa. This can result in dryness and less lubrication, which can make sex uncomfortable. In these cases, the pain is caused by increased friction from the lack of lubrication. Decrease the friction with increased lubrication, and the pain with intercourse goes away. However, atrophy alone does not generally cause true pain. If lubrication is the only issue treated, then the true underlying condition causing the pain isn't addressed, and the pain persists.

ANATOMY

Before we can fully understand any of the individual causes of pain, I think we have to understand something about anatomy. I spend a lot of time explaining this to patients in my office. I believe that if you understand how the vagina develops in the fetus, it is easier to understand the different tissues, the problems associated with them, and their solutions.

Once you appreciate that the vagina is really composed of three different types of tissue, you can see how there can be a number of different problems, each of which has a different solution. There are three divisions to the vagina that are pertinent to our discussions: the vulva, the vestibule, and the vagina.

The Vulva: If you are standing in front of a mirror and you do not touch anything, you are looking at the vulva. It includes the mons pubis (the tissue over the pubic bone), the labia majora (the big lips), the clitoris, and part of the labia minora (the small lips). The vulva extends from what you can see in the mirror to Hart's line, which is about halfway in on the labia minora (the smaller inner lips). Hart's line divides the vulva from the vestibule.

The Vestibule: The vestibule goes from Hart's line to just inside the remnant of the hymen. If you separate the labia majora and the labia minora, you will see Hart's line about halfway in on the labia minora. You can easily see this in most women. If you use a mirror, you can see it for yourself. There is a distinct change in the color of the tissue, from a more consistent flesh tone to a deeper pink or even red. Many women attribute the redness to irritation or infection, but in fact, it is the natural change in the tissue; the change in color is normal. The interlabial sulcus (the space between the labia minor and labia majora) is often redder than the rest of the tissue as well; this, too, does not mean it is inflamed or infected. This is important to know, because if you look at yourself and you see this change in the tissue color and you are having pain, it is easy to assume that this "red" tissue is the problem when, in fact, it is not.

The Vagina: After the vestibule comes the vagina. The vagina starts from just inside the remnant of the hymen and extends to the cervix or the vaginal cuff (if you have had a hysterectomy).

To summarize—from the hair-bearing tissue to Hart's line is the vulva, from Hart's line to just inside the remnant of the hymen is the vestibule, and the rest of the way in toward the uterus is the vagina. The reason I am making this distinction is that these three parts of the female genitalia have different tissues of origin. I know that for most of you, these terms won't mean anything, but I hope they will help you understand the importance of the differences in treating these disorders.

The vulva comes from embryonic tissue called ectoderm, which is the same layer that all of your skin comes from. This is why they have similar characteristics. The vulva is hair-bearing and has sweat and oil glands, etc. It is, for the most part, a dry tissue, similar to the rest of your skin.

The vestibule comes from the primitive urogenital sinus, which is an endoderm germ layer. In fact, the female vestibule is analogous (similar) to the male urethra in development. As such, it has similar characteristics and glands. The vestibule is androgen (male hormone) dependent: this tissue needs both estrogen and testosterone.

The vagina comes from mesoderm and is estrogen dependent. This is why as women get older and experience some vaginal drying, vaginal estrogen can be helpful.

To recap, the vagina comes from mesoderm and needs estrogen, the vestibule comes from the urogenital sinus (endoderm) and needs estrogen and testosterone, and the vulva comes from ectoderm and needs neither estrogen nor testosterone. Later, when we get to the individual disorders and their treatments, having a basic understanding of these different tissues will help you see how important this distinction is.

ANATOMIC SOURCES OF PAIN WITH INTERCOURSE

Pain with intercourse, or dyspareunia, can have three anatomical locations of origin:

1. Introital (entry)
2. Vaginal
3. Pelvic

Introital pain is at the point of insertion and accounts for 80 percent of patients who complain of pain with intercourse. Vaginal pain is pain that comes from the vagina itself, past the entry, and up to the cuff or cervix. Some common causes of pain in the vagina can include things like vaginal dryness or scarring. Pelvic pain (pain with deep thrusting) generally comes from a source in the pelvis outside of the vagina, not necessarily the vagina itself. The pelvic floor muscles, which support the pelvis and surround the vagina, are a common source of this type of pain.

Now that we know a little about the anatomy, let's discuss the different sources of pain. Identifying the location of your pain is critical in order to determine the potential cause. If you were to visit me in my office, I would ask you to describe your pain, and I would then look for clues as to where your pain is coming from. There are several questions I would ask you to help sort this out. I've included these questions below for your reference. It's my hope that these questions will get you to start thinking about your pain.

Knowing where your pain is really coming from is half the battle, so think about your experience as you read the following questions. Your answers to these questions will help you identify the source of your pain so you can better describe it to your doctor—this will help them help you.

1. Does it hurt when the penis first enters the vagina? Or is the pain deeper inside?
2. Do you have problems with speculum exams and tampons?
3. Has it always been painful, or did you once have enjoyable sex that has since become more painful?

4. Since the pain began, have you had some pain-free periods of time, or has the pain been continuous?
5. Did it happen suddenly or come on gradually?
6. Is it in one position or all positions?
7. Do you have pain with clitoral stimulation?
8. Have you ever had what you would consider to be an allergic reaction to a cream used in the vagina?
9. Have you ever had a vaginal infection (yeast or bacterial)?
10. Do you have any bleeding with intercourse?
11. Have you ever had any lesions or sores?
12. Would you describe the pain as burning, tearing, cutting, or ripping? Or is it more aching, throbbing, cramping, or pressure?
13. Does it occur during or after sex?
14. Do you have bladder-related symptoms like increased frequency or urgency? Or do you experience burning during urination?

The answers to these questions can provide very important clues about the cause of your pain.

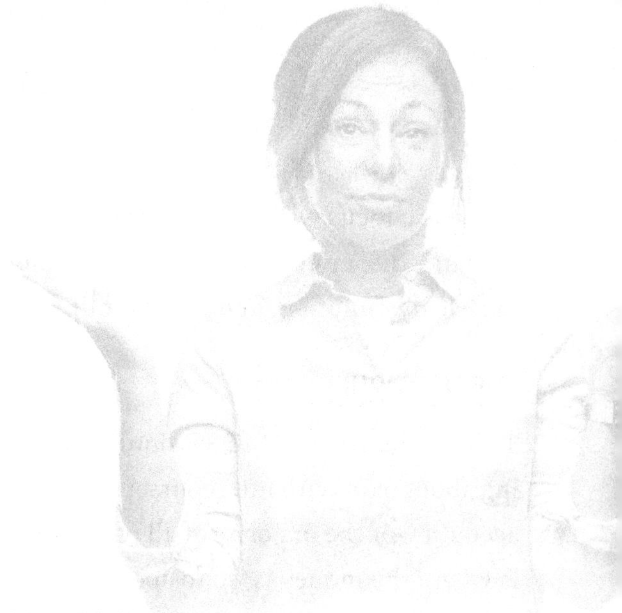

CHAPTER 3

WHAT'S CAUSING THE PAIN?

DIFFERENTIAL DIAGNOSIS FOR INTROITAL PAIN (PAIN ON INSERTION)

As mentioned, the most frequently reported pain associated with intercourse is pain on insertion. There are a variety of causes of this pain, including:

1. Hormonally Mediated Vestibulodynia (most common cause)
2. Hypertonic Pelvic Floor Muscle Dysfunction (second most common cause)
3. Neuroproliferative Vestibulodynia—too many nerve endings (third most common cause)
4. Lichen Sclerosus or Lichen Planus

Our main focus will be on the top three most common causes of introital pain—hormonally mediated vestibulodynia, hypertonic pelvic floor muscle dysfunction, and neuroproliferative vestibulodynia.

THE VESTIBULE

The vestibule is the MOST significant part of our anatomy when talking about pain with intercourse, so it deserves a bit more detail here—it accounts for the majority of all pain women have with intercourse! This is where the money is, so to speak.

As mentioned earlier, the vestibule is derived from tissue that is very similar to the male urethra. It has a different blood supply than the vagina, which is important because many women are given vaginal estrogen for atrophy, but the vestibule needs estrogen too. Because the blood supply is different, any estrogen inserted into the vagina does not help the vestibule. So, if you have used Vagifem or Estring, you were not getting any estrogen to the vestibule, only the vagina. You must apply some estrogen directly to the vestibule for it to benefit from such treatment. This is why, in my opinion, creams (Estrace and Premarin) are better for treating vaginal atrophy.

The vestibule also has several very important glands. These glands are **the most common causes of pain** in women. Right next to the urethra, on either side, are the Skene glands and the minor vestibular glands. The Skene glands are similar to the male prostate, and the minor vestibular glands are similar to the glands found in men called the Littre glands. Although very rare, women can develop a cancer in these glands that is very similar to prostate cancer.

It's important to note that these are androgen-dependent glands. That means they **need testosterone**! Without testosterone, these glands do not work well, and they become clogged, not unlike a clogged pore on your face that then develops into a tender pimple. When this happens to these glands, you can see why it would hurt when they are touched.

The Skene and minor vestibular glands are located next to the urethra at positions 1 and 11 o'clock. On the back wall of the vestibule are more glands, called the Bartholin glands or the major vestibular glands. These glands are on the back side of the introitus (entry to the vagina) at the 5 and 7 o'clock positions. They are similar to the Cowper glands in men, which are testosterone-dependent, mucin-secreting glands. So, the Bartholin glands also need testosterone; without it, they too become unhealthy and, therefore, painful.

HORMONALLY MEDIATED VESTIBULODYNIA

Since the majority of cases of pain during sex can be attributed to the vestibule, most of you reading this will find your answers here. The number one cause of vestibule pain with intercourse is hormonally mediated vestibulodynia.

In fact, the young lady I described earlier, Debbie, had hormonally mediated vestibulodynia. It is a common condition in young women who are on birth control pills and in older women who are on oral estrogen replacements. That's right—birth control pills can cause this condition! Most women will describe previously having a normal sex life. They enjoyed sex, and it was pain-free. Then, after starting birth control pills, sex gradually became painful.

BCPs and Vestibulodynia

Birth control pills (BCPs)—the most common medication prescribed for young women—were directly responsible for causing Debbie's problem. Ironically, many women start BCPs so they can enjoy sex without worrying about the consequence of an unwanted pregnancy. Yet the very thing that helped them have responsible sex then destroys their sex life!

If you have pain with sex and you are taking birth control pills, then it's likely that you have hormonally mediated vestibulodynia and should seriously consider a non-hormonal form of birth control. A diaphragm or IUD would be nice alternatives to consider.

Here are some statistics. According to Dr. Irwin Goldstein, Director of Sexual Medicine at Alvarado Hospital and Clinical Professor of Surgery at University of California at San Diego, studies show that women who use BCPs before the age of seventeen have a 920 percent greater chance of developing vestibulodynia (pain in the vestibule) than women who have never used BCPs. And women who start after age 17 have a 460 percent greater chance of developing vestibulodynia than someone who has never used BCPs. Once you develop hormonally mediated vestibulodynia, it can be difficult to reverse. Unfortunately, while stopping the birth control pills will help, it may not completely solve the problem.

I think that all women should engage in responsible sexual activity and avoid unwanted pregnancies. I personally was on BCPs for eighteen years, and I loved the convenience of them. But in this conversation, they are likely not your friend. I would recommend trying a diaphragm or talking to your doctor about an IUD. This will allow your hormones to go back to normal. However, this is a personal decision you will need to make. For those of you on an oral estrogen replacement, like Premarin, talk to your doctor about changing to a topical form.

So, why do birth control pills increase the chances of developing vestibulodynia? We all have both estrogen and testosterone. They are normal hormones in both men and women, although in different proportions. For men, testosterone is the dominant hormone, but they have and need estrogen too. Estrogen helps prevent cardiovascular disease and osteoporosis in men.

In women, estrogen is the dominant hormone, but we have and need some testosterone as well. The vestibular glands are dependent on testosterone, and so is our libido (sex drive). When our testosterone levels are low, we experience a lot of the same symptoms that men with diminished testosterone levels do, including low libido, low energy, and trouble achieving orgasm.

Problems occur when estrogen and testosterone levels are out of balance. When we take any form of estrogen by mouth, be it BCPs or oral estrogen replacement after menopause, this balance is upset. Levels of free testosterone drop, which means the vestibular glands do not have enough testosterone to function normally. They become unhealthy, and you end up with vestibulodynia and painful intercourse.

Vestibulodynia does not just happen to young women on BCPs. We know that as we near menopause, we make less estrogen. But as women get older, they naturally make less testosterone as well. There is very little mention of this in the medical community, but this decrease in testosterone has significant implications for us women. If women take oral estrogen for replacement to relieve the symptoms of menopause, the problem may be exacerbated. The result can be even lower free testosterone levels, leading to vestibulodynia. Fortunately, not all women who go through menopause will have problems with low testosterone, but many do, and hormone replacement can make it more likely.

Are Your Symptoms From Vestibulodynia?

The information that follows is not meant to be used for self-diagnosis or in place of a professional medical assessment. Rather, these details are intended to help you think about and more accurately identify the source of your pain, in order to help you have a more productive dialogue with your healthcare provider.

Vestibulodynia simply means pain in the vestibule. The pain in this condition comes from unhealthy vestibular glands, located in the vestibule between the labia minora and the remnant of the hymen at 1, 3, 5, 6, 7, 9, and 11 o'clock. You can try to identify these glands yourself with a mirror and a cotton swab. Separate the labia majora and minora so you can see the entry to the vagina. Identify the opening of the urethra. Start there and gently touch yourself on either side of the urethra with a moistened cotton swab. Does this replicate the pain that you have with intercourse?

Then, gently touch the other vestibular glands that go around the entry in the positions listed above. If they are all tender, then you most likely have hormonally mediated vestibulodynia. These mucin-secreting glands become unhealthy and do not function normally, becoming clogged with debris, bacteria, and sloughing cells. As a result, they become tender to the touch. Women with vestibulodynia will have pain with penetration during intercourse. Speculum exams at the gynecologist's office are also painful. Even the use of a tampon may be too much for some women. In severe cases, it can be painful just to sit for long periods of time.

One word of caution: If the glands at 5, 6, and 7 o'clock are tender, but the ones next to the urethra are not, then this is not your diagnosis. In that case, you likely have a *hypertonic pelvic floor*, which I will discuss next.

Treating Hormonally Mediated Vestibulodynia

I know that at this point, things may sound very depressing. You once had an enjoyable sex life. Then, you started BCPs to avoid an unwanted pregnancy (very responsible, by the way), or you started oral estrogen replacement to counteract the symptoms of menopause. This resulted in lower levels of free testosterone, causing your vestibular glands to shut down and become unhealthy, which led to the pain you are now having.

Somehow, you have to get testosterone back to the glands so they can function normally again. Because women who are taking any form of oral estrogen experience low free testosterone levels, the first thing you need to do is stop the oral estrogen!

Women on birth control pills should find an alternative method of birth control, and menopausal women on oral estrogen should switch to a topical form of estrogen. You can switch to a compounded form of estrogen, a patch, or a commercially available estrogen, like Evamist. Once you stop the oral estrogen, you will need to be patient. It takes time for balance to be restored sufficiently to reduce symptoms and pain. This is going to be difficult for some of you and should not be taken lightly.

There are a couple of ways you can begin to restore testosterone to the proper level. You can apply topical cream to the glands, or it can be achieved systemically, with a testosterone preparation absorbed into the bloodstream through the skin. Everyone with hormonally mediated vestibulodynia can use a topical estradiol/testosterone cream directly on the glands, regardless of the cause. So, whether you are a young woman on BCPs or a postmenopausal woman with low total testosterone levels, you can treat the glands locally. If you use the topical cream, you apply it to the glands twice a day until the pain goes away.

For the second method, testosterone preparations that are absorbed through the skin, you can use either a commercially available form of testosterone or a compounded testosterone that can be made for you at a compounding pharmacy. I generally prescribe compounded formulations in my practice because it is easy to customize them to each woman's needs, and they can be combined with estrogen and progesterone, if appropriate.

The commercially available form of testosterone that I use most often is Testim because I think it is the easiest product for women to use. All of the pharmaceutical testosterone supplements are packaged for men, so the quantities are too high for women, who need one-tenth of the amount of testosterone that men do. Testim comes in a little tube that can be recapped, which makes this ideal for women. A man would use one tube per day while a woman will use one tube over ten days. The bottom line is you need to replace your testosterone just like men do. I will give you more information about this later.

There is also an oral supplement that can be taken to help raise your natural testosterone levels: DHEA. This can be found at any drug store or nutrition store. DHEA is the precursor to testosterone, meaning your body uses DHEA to make testosterone. The evidence for how well this works on its own is weak, however. But it is easy to get because it is sold over the counter and might be worth a try.

Whether you supplement your testosterone topically (as a cream applied directly on the glands) or systemically (by raising serum testosterone levels), the glands will start to heal. But either way will take time—the longer it's been going on, the longer it will take to reverse the condition. Do not expect to see significant improvement in the first six weeks. Although I have seen symptoms begin to improve within as little as two weeks, this is not the norm. About 50 percent of women will see

Another Negative Contribution of BCPs

Another way that BCPs contribute to the development of pain with intercourse is that they cause a change in the structure of the vaginal mucosa, which consists of a top layer called the epithelium and a deeper layer called the lamina propria. The dermal papillae connect the two and look like waves of finger-like projections between them.

There is a morphological change in the pattern of the dermal papillae (a layer under the surface) that occurs in women on BCPs. These finger-like projections become much flatter. This flattening reduces the ability of the underlying layer of the vaginal wall to interlock with the epithelium (the top layer), making the top layer more sensitive to mechanical stress or strain. So, with the back and forth motion of intercourse, the top layer will shear away from the papillae, and you will get micro-tears in the mucosa. Ouch! This change in the vaginal mucosa happens within a few months of starting BCPs. Sorry to be the bearer of such bad news. I, too, loved my BCPs. But as I look back on my own sex life, I can see how BCPs negatively affected me. It all makes sense to me now. I just wish I had known what I was doing to myself. Hopefully, you can learn from this information and make better choices than I did and return to a rich and fulfilling sex life.

improvement at twelve weeks, but it can take up to six months, so be patient and consistent.

Menopause and Other Causes of Hormonally Mediated Vestibulodynia

There are other causes of vestibulodynia besides BCPs. These include natural menopause, surgical removal of the ovaries, hormonal control of endometriosis or hirsutism, breastfeeding, infertility treatments, hormone manipulation for the treatment of breast cancer, or any manipulation of hormones for any reason.

Medications like spironolactone, commonly used for the treatment of hirsutism or acne, can cause vestibulodynia because they block testosterone receptors. Tamoxifen and aromatase inhibitors (Arimidex, Femara, and Aromasin), commonly used in the treatment of breast cancer, are other culprits.

Tamoxifen is the worst of these because it actually binds to and poisons the receptor. With the aromatase inhibitors, you can still treat the glands directly with low dose estrogen and testosterone creams, which will get rid of the pain and allow you to still stay on the aromatase inhibitor. Unfortunately, this does not work for women on Tamoxifen. In order for topical treatments to work, they will have to change to one of the aromatase inhibitors.

HYPERTONIC PELVIC FLOOR

The second most common cause of pain with intercourse is having a hypertonic pelvic floor. This means you have pelvic floor spasms. Any muscle can go into spasms. You have probably experienced a charley horse before; if so, you can appreciate how painful a muscle spasm can be. Increased tension in muscles causes a decrease in blood flow, which then decreases the oxygen supply to the muscles. This leads to a buildup of lactic acid, especially at the point where the muscle connects to the bone. A ten percent increase in muscle tension decreases blood flow by 50 percent. That is huge!

Most women with a hypertonic pelvic floor have an increased tension of 40–50 percent, so their decrease in blood flow is easily 80–90 percent. This results in a significant increase in lactic acid levels and causes muscle pain, especially at the ends of the pelvic floor muscles (levator ani) that are in the vagina at the back of the introitus. This also causes superficial tenderness on the back side of the entry to the vagina (or vestibule), which in turn causes pain on entry to the vagina with particular discomfort on the back side of the vagina.

The overlying mucosa will seem tender, but it is the underlying tense muscle that is causing the problem. The mucosa may also be red in appearance. Since the pelvic floor muscles are in spasms, most women (though not all) will also have pain along the sidewalls of the vagina that presents with deeper penetration. Essentially, with a hypertonic pelvic floor, you can have pain at the entry to the vagina and also deeper within.

Muscles of the Pelvic Floor

What's the connection between pelvic floor muscles and painful sex? Everything's connected. Your pelvic organs rest on a shelf of muscles collectively called the levator ani muscles, which pass the rectum, the vagina, and the urethra. These muscles attach at the entry of the vagina along the back wall. For people with hypertonic pelvic floor issues, several muscles can be involved in this scenario, and any (or all of them) can be in spasm, contributing to your pain.

The coccyges muscles are deep in the vagina on either side. If these muscles are in spasms, they will cause two types of pain. The first is in the muscle itself. The second is at the entry of the vagina. This is why I told you earlier that if the vestibular glands are only tender along the back side, it is not hormonally mediated vestibulodynia but hypertonic pelvic floor. If these muscles are in spasm, it will be painful to touch them anywhere along the muscle. Your pain will be present with pressure on the muscle deep inside and on entry. You can often feel a band where the muscles are in spasm. It will, of course, also hurt when you press on them.

Jill's Story

Jill's story is a little different. She came to see me with a number of complaints. She, too, was a successful young businesswoman with a career that was advancing and rewarding. She was single and sexually active. I could tell from the first few minutes with her that she was a real go-getter—driven and focused. She had what I would call a Type A personality. She was also physically fit. She exercised regularly (yoga and Pilates).

Her primary complaints centered on her bladder. She was getting up several times at night and urinating more frequently during the day. When asked, she also admitted to being constipated. She had a normal sex life that had slowly become more painful. She described pain on entry, but also a deeper pain that felt like it involved the whole pelvis. She did not describe it as burning but rather more as a strong achy pain or really strong pressure. The pain endured after sex as well. She described heaviness, throbbing, and a tightness in her pelvis.

During her exam, the vestibular glands near the urethra were normal, although the glands on the back part of the vestibule were tender and even inflamed. When I examined her pelvic floor muscles along the walls of the vagina, she wanted to jump off the exam table. They were tight and rigid. Jill had the second most common cause of pain with intercourse: a hypertonic pelvic floor. With proper treatment, she is now pain-free.

Symptoms of Hypertonic Pelvic Floor

A hypertonic pelvic floor can cause a wide range of symptoms. While pain with intercourse is one of them, there are many others. See if any of these describe you.

Generalized vulvar pain or burning. I have had patients who experienced constant pain, not just during intercourse. It was uncomfortable and painful to sit or wear tight pants. The tenderness we discussed where the muscles attach is a likely cause for this constant pain. It is also why it hurts with penetration and can generate an even deeper pain.

Urinary complaints about frequency, urgency, hesitancy, or incomplete emptying. Constipation, hemorrhoids, and rectal fissures can develop as well. A hypertonic pelvic floor is often associated with holding urine. We call it "nurse's bladder" (or "teacher's bladder" in my office), but anyone who delays voiding for any reason can develop a hypertonic pelvic floor.

Excessive abdominal strengthening exercises. Women or men who are avid about abdominal strengthening exercises are prone to developing pelvic floor spasms. Pilates and yoga instructors are particularly vulnerable. They may get a strong core, but the price could also be a hypertonic pelvic floor and pain with intercourse.

Type A personalities. Women with a lot of anxiety or stress are more likely to develop a hypertonic pelvic floor. This is one more reason why we Type A personality women (yes, I am one of them too) need to get ourselves under control. We all have stress, and we all manage it differently. Unfortunately, we often harbor our stress in some manner in our bodies. Women are far more likely to do this in the pelvis than men, who tend to see the ill effects of stress in the upper body, like the chest, neck, and back areas.

There are no universal rules about this observation. It is just my own observation. I believe one of the reasons women manifest stress in the pelvis is that this is the seat of our femininity. It is where we conceive and carry our children. It is our center. It is our core. But the reason is not really important. The manifestation of our stress as something physical and painful is what really matters. With stress, we tend to tighten muscles, and when we do this chronically, these muscles can go into spasm. Nothing good comes from poorly managed stress!

Other conditions that can predispose you to hypertonic pelvic floor issues include scoliosis, sacroiliac joint dysfunction, piriformis syndrome, low back pain, and hip/labral tears. Any of these can cause tightening of the pelvic floor muscles, which then go into spasm and ultimately lead to painful intercourse.

A Word on the Term Vaginismus

Vaginismus is an outdated term that has been removed from the *American Psychiatric Association's Diagnostic and Statistical Manual of Mental Disorders* (DSM-5). It was removed from this authoritative guide because listing it there suggested a psychological cause for the problem, which there is not. Vaginismus is a very real physical problem. Unfortunately, many women, maybe even you, have been told that it is a voluntary tightening of the muscles. In other words, you just need to relax. If you have been told this, I am sorry! Let me assure you that this is not your fault.

The good news is that it is treatable. We often use physical therapy to break the tension in pelvic floor muscles. We also sometimes prescribe medications, like muscle relaxants (e.g., low dose valium taken by mouth) or compound creams that are applied directly to the muscles vaginally.

More Than One Cause of Dyspareunia

It is not uncommon to have both hormonally mediated vestibulodynia and a hypertonic pelvic floor. The reason for this is that once you have pain from any cause, your pelvic floor muscles will tighten in response and then may go into spasm. This is why I talked about the cycle of pain earlier. You can see how this can be a very complicated problem that is not always easy to sort out!

Treating a Hypertonic Pelvic Floor

If the discussion of hypertonic pelvic floor resonates with you and you feel that this may be your problem, what can you do about it? Well, like any other muscle spasm, you need to break the spasm and get the muscle to relax. There are several ways to do this. First, if stress is part of the problem, you need to get a handle on it. Find a healthy outlet for your stress and learn to relax your mind and body. Hot baths, meditation, and heating pads can all be very helpful when consistently used. In an effort to break the spasm cycle, I may prescribe muscle relaxants on a short-term basis.

The mainstay for treating pelvic floor spasms, though, is physical therapy. You need to find a physical therapist who is specifically trained in this area and have them work with you to break the muscle spasm. You can find an appropriately trained physical therapist in your area by going to either APTAPelvicHealth.org or HermanWallace.com.

You may augment physical therapy with other treatments (such as Botox injections, trigger point injections, biofeedback, and vaginal dilators) to help slowly stretch the muscles. Vaginal dilators can be particularly helpful for older women who have developed tight vaginal openings or shortened vaginas after vaginal surgery. In the latter case, you may need to soften the mucosa with vaginal estrogen to optimize the vaginal dilator's effectiveness. Vaginal estrogen is a prescription you can easily get from your primary care doctor if you are postmenopausal.

NEUROPROLIFERATIVE VESTIBULODYNIA

Neuroproliferative vestibulodynia is the third most common cause of pain and occurs when you have too many pain receptors (C-afferent nociceptors) in the vaginal mucosa. As a result, you experience pain any time the tissue is touched. Even wearing certain clothes, like jeans, can cause some women extreme discomfort. You can be born with too many pain receptors, or you can develop them following repeated infections or allergic reactions.

In healthy women, these receptors are located below what is called the basement membrane of the mucosa. The excess release of substances from mast cells (as can happen with infections or allergic reactions) stimulates these receptors to multiply and grow. When they do this, they break through the basement membrane and lie closer to the surface. In turn, this can also cause your body to develop too many of them—up to thirty times the normal number of these pain receptors. The result of so many pain receptors is intense pain in the entire vestibule, not just the vestibular glands. The pain is typically located from Hart's line to just inside the remnant of the hymen.

The congenital version is something with which you are born and have likely been managing throughout your life. It is also part of a larger syndrome. In fact, sixty percent of people with congenital neuroproliferative vestibulodynia will also have very sensitive belly buttons. If you have always had pain in the vestibule along with a sensitive belly button, then this might be your problem.

Far more common, however, is acquired neuroproliferative vestibulodynia. Women usually report the onset of these symptoms after a severe yeast infection, recurrent yeast infections, or an allergic reaction to a cream used to treat a vaginal infection. Women who develop this are genetically predisposed to developing this condition.

However, there are treatment options. If you have experienced symptoms for less than six months, you can usually be treated medically with interferon, which stabilizes the cells causing the problem. If it has been going on for more than six months, some topical treatments can help. Topical lidocaine preparations can decrease pain and discomfort.

These can be purchased over-the-counter or with a prescription. Be very careful if you try over-the-counter versions. Sometimes the ointment base (what the lidocaine is combined with) can cause a reaction, so go gently on a small area to start. Generally, a cream is better than a gel. Gabapentin and desipramine are two other medications that can help, but they require a prescription.

If topical treatments fail, then you may need to see someone who can surgically excise the vestibule. Keep in mind that surgery is rarely the solution for most patients. Of the 500 patients who are seen each year at the San Diego Sexual Medicine clinic (an excellent place to go if you are on the West Coast), only seven percent are candidates for this surgery. While surgery is not done frequently, it has a cure rate in up to 71 percent of patients who have failed other regimens.

Finding a surgeon with experience is the hard part. I recommend looking at the International Society for the Study of Women's Sexual Health (ISSWSH) website for a directory of surgeons in your area—ISSWSH.org. This specialized resource provides the highest likelihood of finding someone trained in this procedure.

When you call for an appointment, ask if the surgeon performs vestibulectomies before putting too much of your time and effort into it. If this is your diagnosis, then you probably have already seen too many doctors who could not help you. While I do not perform this surgery myself, if you have trouble finding someone in your area, send me an email. Perhaps I can help you locate someone.

OTHER DISORDERS

Although I have addressed the most common causes of pain with intercourse, a few words on some other conditions are warranted.

Lichen Sclerosus and Lichen Planus

There are some dermatologic conditions that can cause pain (though more commonly itching) of the vulva. Lichen sclerosus and lichen planus are two skin conditions that affect the vulva. They both have a whitish appearance to them, and a biopsy is required to confirm the diagnosis. Once correctly identified, they can be treated with steroids.

Lichen sclerosus can cause phimosis of the clitoral hood. Phimosis is something most commonly attributed to uncircumcised men whose foreskin gets too tight to retract. Just as the penis has a foreskin, so does the clitoris. This foreskin, or hood, needs to be able to retract. If this tissue becomes scarred, it may no longer be able to retract to expose the clitoris.

If you have difficulty reaching orgasm with clitoral stimulation or you have a lot of pain or itching at the clitoris, then you may have phimosis. Check by trying to retract the hood. It should easily pull back to reveal the clitoris underneath. If you cannot do this directly or with a mirror, then have your partner or someone you trust help you. If it does not retract, see a medical professional. Treatment typically begins with topical steroids, and if those do not work, it can be surgically corrected.

Vaginal Atrophy

Vaginal atrophy is a very common and problematic issue. It involves the thinning, inflammation, and drying of the vaginal walls and occurs when your body has less estrogen. This typically happens after menopause and can make intercourse painful. I did not address this earlier because anyone who has complained to their doctor about pain with intercourse is likely to be prescribed vaginal estrogen. However, if that was the only component of your pain, the problem would have been solved, and you would not have been drawn to read this book.

Low Estrogen

Let me take a brief aside here. I am a big supporter of the use of estrogen—systemic or vaginal. It was not that long ago that our ovaries lasted as long as we needed them. The average life expectancy one hundred years ago was about the life expectancy of our ovaries. Now, we live almost as long post-menopause, but for some reason, we are expected to live with all the ramifications of low hormone levels! To me, that does not make any sense. If your thyroid is low, we replace that; if you have poor insulin function, we treat that too. Just because something happens as a result of aging does not mean you should have to live with it.

I believe the Women's Health Initiative study done in 2002 has done a huge disservice to women. The results were grossly misreported in the media, and as a result, many women and physicians falsely believe that estrogen is universally bad. That is unfortunate.

If you have vaginal dryness, there is a safe and effective treatment for this. Many studies have shown that vaginal estrogen does not get absorbed into your circulation to any significant degree. So even if you do not want systemic estrogen because of breast or ovarian cancer concerns, it is safe to use vaginally. Also, the doses are very small. For example, an entire year's supply of Vagifem does not equal the dose of one oral tablet of estrogen.

There are also other alternatives you may consider. For instance, a compounded DHEA can be used. It is not estrogen, but the vaginal mucosa uses it as estrogen. It must be compounded by a compounding pharmacy, but it is fairly easy to get. There is also a medicine called Osphena, which is an oral tablet. It is not estrogen but has an estrogen-like effect on vaginal mucosa, thickening it just like estrogen without having to take any estrogen. This can be prescribed by your primary doctor as well.

Lubrication

This is another topic that deserves some discussion in relation to vaginal atrophy. Lack of estrogen causes vaginal atrophy, which then leads to a thinning of the vaginal mucosa and vaginal dryness. These changes lead to insufficient lubrication during intercourse, which will then be uncomfortable for two reasons. One, the lack of lubrication causes increased friction, which pulls on the mucosa. Two, the thinner mucosa cannot handle the tension on it because of changes in its structure, and you will get a sheering or separation of the top layer off of the basement membrane. So vaginal atrophy, if present, should be treated. It is very common with aging and can happen any time after we start having hormonal changes, as early as age thirty-five.

Here are a few final thoughts about treating vaginal atrophy. First, vaginal dryness comes from a lack of estrogen, so consider using something either topically or orally. Additional lubrication can be helpful. You can use lubricants at the time of intercourse, or you can use vaginal moisturizers, which will adhere to the vaginal mucosa for two to three days at a time. Some good moisturizers I recommend are Refresh, Replens, and K-Y Pearls. There are lots of lubricants available at your local pharmacy.

Make sure you are using something that is water-based and not petroleum-based. Do NOT use Vaseline. The brand I typically recommend is Astroglide, but there are several for you to try. Experiment with them and find the one that you like the best. There are two other natural lubricants that I recommend to my patients: olive oil and coconut oil. They are both natural oils that you can easily find and work very nicely for this purpose. Again, experiment and find what works best for you.

Scarring

Surgeries often result in residual scarring. After a hysterectomy, for instance, you can get some shortening of the vagina and scarring at the cuff. With the repair of a fallen bladder, you can get more scarring, narrowing, or shortening of the vagina. Women who are not sexually active will also experience a shortening and tightening of the vagina from lack of use—the "use it or lose it" principle does apply here. Sometimes the introitus (opening) can get too tight for penetration, or the length of the vagina can be too short for adequate penetration during intercourse, and this can cause pain.

These problems are harder to fix, but a combination of vaginal estrogen and vaginal dilators can be very helpful. I recommend "cool water cones," which you can easily find on the internet for cheap. Using these daily while nourishing the vagina mucosa with estrogen will slowly help stretch and loosen the tissue to work up to intercourse.

CHAPTER 4

NEW TREATMENTS

I HAVE SPENT MUCH OF MY CAREER treating problems with prescriptions and surgery. However, modern medicine continues to search for new treatments, and some recent technological advances show promise in treating female sexual dysfunction. Specifically, these advances target how to help the body heal itself. Many people want less invasive, more natural solutions to fix physical ailments, and I am happy to say that these solutions are now available—pill-free and surgery-free solutions to better health.

THE ANSWER TO YOUR PRAYERS

In my practice, I only use safe, proven solutions to treat symptoms of gynecological issues, including pain, dysfunction, and incontinence. Two relatively recent therapeutic treatment options that I've added to my practice are platelet-rich plasma (PRP) therapy and radiofrequency technology.

These methods are effective at treating various vaginal-related problems, including eliminating incontinence, reducing or eliminating painful intercourse, reducing vaginal laxity, and enhancing sexual responsiveness.

PLATELET-RICH PLASMA THERAPY

Platelet-rich plasma (PRP) therapy has been used in many areas of medicine. It has proven to be a natural way of letting your body heal itself and involves injecting a high concentration of platelet-rich plasma, derived from a patient's own blood, into the affected or injured area of the body.

I am certified in a form of PRP therapy you may have heard of called the O-Shot®. The procedure is a form of PRP therapy that is effective in the treatment of incontinence as well as other gynecological problems.

The O-Shot was developed by Charles Runels, MD, when he observed that there were a growing number of women in his practice who experienced incontinence, decreased sex drive, vaginal dryness from menopause or breast cancer treatment, painful intercourse, and the inability to orgasm.

Dr. Runels began to perceive female sexuality as a holistic and dynamic structure, referring to it as "The Female Orgasm System." This phrase came out of the need to think about female sexuality with the same elegance, detail, and utility as is used for the other systems of the body. A woman's sexual response and health are just as intricate as the endocrine system or the nervous system. If the health of her orgasm system is taken seriously, each female has the capacity for orgasm and sexual fulfillment.

Over the past 20 years, researchers have been looking at ways to extract growth factors from the bloodstream. It's known that these growth factors stimulate wound healing. Whenever there is an injury to tissue, the body activates and releases platelets, and a whole host of growth factors go to work to restore that tissue back to health. You might remember watching a scraped knee heal when you were young. These platelets and growth factors made that healing possible.

In addition to healing injuries, these same elements have been found to promote healing from disease or after surgery. For example, studies have demonstrated that putting this platelet-rich plasma into a damaged knee can help regenerate cartilage.

HOW THE O-SHOT WORKS

The procedure is simple. First, a woman's own blood is drawn from her arm. FDA-approved equipment is used to separate the platelet-rich plasma from the blook. This natural substance contains all of the growth factors that are responsible for healing. The process is safe! Medical research shows no reports of serious side effects from PRP therapy when prepared using FDA-approved equipment, and about 20 different machines for this purpose have been approved by the FDA.

After the patient's PRP is separated out, the provider helps the patient apply a numbing cream to the areas near her clitoris and inside her vagina. When numb, the PRP is injected using a thin needle (the same size used in the face and mouth with cosmetic procedures). Approximately one teaspoon of PRP is injected into the roof of the vagina, and one-fifth of a teaspoon goes into the clitoris. Most women do not experience any pain during the procedure.

When PRP is injected between the vaginal wall and the urethra, the healing process begins. New fibroblasts infiltrate the tissue and are activated. The vaginal epithelium is restored to a healthier state. It thickens and becomes better lubricated. This thickening is also what supports the tissue under the urethra, which helps to eliminate incontinence. As a result, sensation during intercourse is improved, and libido naturally increases.

The healing effects take hold within hours of getting the shot and continue to improve for up to six months. It's been reported that a second shot administered about three months later will prolong and improve the benefits even more.

Over 90 percent of women injected with the O-Shot show a marked decrease in their incontinence symptoms. It can also provide dramatic improvements for women who experience pain with intercourse or the inability to be aroused and/or reach orgasm.

After receiving the O-Shot, one woman reported, *"That shot changed my life! I've lost weight, and I'm not depressed because I can sleep and exercise. I think having orgasms makes me less anxious and depressed. I'm a better mother, and I'm doing better at the bank, just because I feel so much better."* Her urinary incontinence was no longer a problem, and she was sleeping through the night. This allowed her to get back to jogging and walking daily for exercise, which significantly improved her mood. Anxiety was no longer an issue, and she could have comfortable sex—all from a shot that took 15 minutes over her lunch hour!

My Personal Experience

I want to share my own story with you because I believe it helps all of us if we speak about the problems we are having. By communicating, we can help each other find solutions and know that we're not alone.

I consider myself to be a pretty typical woman who is getting a little older. My desire was waning, and I was starting to have a little pain. It was not as severe as what some of my patients report, but I felt discomfort just the same. I still achieved an orgasm, but not as easily as when I was younger. Sometimes, it seemed like more work than it was worth. Mostly because I wanted to see for myself what the fuss was all about, I tried the O-Shot. The first thing I will tell you is that it did not hurt at all. I mean, not one bit! I was told I could be sexually active right away. My husband was open to the idea and thought we should check it out immediately.

Three days later (again, testing out the O-Shot for research purposes), I had the longest orgasm I have ever had! I did not think it would stop. My pain was also gone.

As a scientist, I admit that I am always a little skeptical about new treatments. But combining solid research with my personal experience, I can confidently give the O-Shot five stars! As I'm writing this section of the book, I am seven months in, and things are still rocking and rolling for my husband and me in the bedroom!

Whether you have problems with urine leakage/incontinence, or you want to reignite the bedroom fires in your relationship and experience incredibly powerful orgasms similar to the pleasure that your partner enjoys, the O-Shot just might be the perfect solution for you!

RADIOFREQUENCY TREATMENT

When collagen and elastin levels decrease, tissues become loose and sag. We know a lot about this phenomenon thanks to all of the face creams that are marketed to us to fight the effects of time. However, this is occurring everywhere in our bodies, and the vagina is affected too. Radiofrequency treatment uses energy to heat deep tissues to a higher temperature in order to stimulate the body to produce collagen.

Radiofrequency treatment of the vagina has been demonstrated to naturally stimulate the production of collagen and elastin, which keeps tissues tight and pliable. There are several radiofrequency treatments available, but the one that I believe is the most therapeutic is called the Viveve® System. It is the only product on the market actively running phase 3 trials with the FDA to demonstrate its clinical efficacy. Additionally, there is an impressive amount of data showing its success in treating incontinence.

About Viveve® System

The Viveve System tightens and strengthens by heating deep tissues. This process uses the company's patented, cryogen-cooled monopolar radiofrequency (CMRF) technology to stimulate collagen production, which reinvigorates tissue. This can be accomplished in just ONE session.

Viveve has been actively working with the FDA over the last two years to address any potential safety concerns and is currently running clinical trials for stress urinary incontinence, under FDA review. Additionally, a Viveve study is being conducted to evaluate a new investigational treatment for women who are having urine leakage or pain during sex following childbirth.

Many women experience anatomical changes to their pelvic anatomy following childbirth. These changes can have a long-term impact on a women's sex life, affecting desire, arousal, and even orgasmic response. Additionally, many women may begin to experience pain with intercourse, changes in sensation/satisfaction, and decreased lubrication.

During a Viveve treatment procedure, the tissue just inside the vagina is treated using radiofrequency (RF) energy to heat the vaginal tissue, while a surface coolant protects the treated tissue. The deep heating targets the connective tissue that plays a role in the structural integrity of the vagina and urinary systems.

The Viveve protocol was modified for sexual function to provide additional energy to the tissue beyond the introitus to support the urethra and improve stress urinary incontinence. Clinical trial results have shown statistically significant and clinically important improvements in sexual arousal, lubrication, and orgasm as an added benefit to curing urinary incontinence.

Via its minimally invasive CMRF therapy, Viveve is proven to safely treat vaginal tissue in women who have reported vaginal laxity and painful intercourse. The treatment enhances the structural integrity of the genito-pelvic-clitoral complex (the mechanism by which we achieve orgasm) by enriched fibroblastic deposited connective tissue. In other words, it remodels the tissue so that sex feels better, and we have better orgasms.

CMRF therapy has been found to alleviate female stress urinary incontinence, but it has also been associated with statistically significant and clinically important improvements in sexual function and pleasure. How's that for an added bonus?

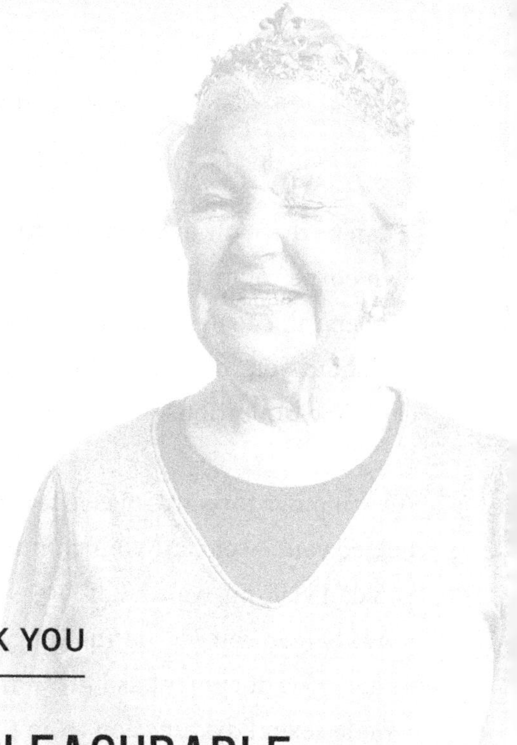

THANK YOU

HERE'S TO A PLEASURABLE AND PAIN-FREE SEX LIFE!

I hope the information I have shared has given you a better understanding of what is going on with your body. When you go to see a physician, I want you to feel confident and informed, knowing that you shouldn't feel awkward or embarrassed to have an honest discussion with your doctor about your concerns.

Effective treatment requires a correct diagnosis, and that is best done by working with your physician. The challenge is that understanding and explaining what is happening with our own bodies can be difficult. Luckily, the field of female sexual dysfunction is rapidly expanding, and our treatment options are expanding as well.

It can be difficult to keep up with changes and innovations (even in our own corner of medicine). I ask you to forgive yourself, anyone who has not been able to help you, and those who have been less than understanding about your difficulty. Remember, we are all human and subject to the same limitations.

As you move forward, please let me know if anything I have shared has helped you. I welcome your comments at DrEisenbrown@gmail.com, or you can visit my website at DrEisenbrown.com. Tell me your story and how I helped you get the answers you were looking for. I will continually update this document as I grow and learn more about the conditions of female sexual dysfunction from the latest research.

If you live in the Orlando area or travel this way and want to talk to me about how this might help you, your partner, and your relationship, feel free to contact me for a consultation to discuss any treatment regimens I've discussed in this book.

Join my mailing list if you want to be kept informed about new information as it becomes available. You can do so easily by texting "sex" to 474747 or by emailing us at Contact@AmoreMedicalSpa.com. You can also learn more about what we are doing on our website: AmoreMedicalSpa.com. I will be writing about lots of other related conditions and would love for you to benefit from it all.

Thank you for taking the time to read what I have to share, and God bless you! I wish you a long and pleasurable sex life!

—Dr. Nicole Eisenbrown

Made in the USA
Monee, IL
04 November 2026

67385551R00030